FLORENCE NIGHTINGALE AT HARLEY STREET

Sir Harry Verney's recent unexpected discovery of the papers in Florence Nightingale's handwriting which are the subject of this volume came at an apt moment as 1970 is the 150th anniversary of her birth. These papers are illuminating quarterly reports to the Governors of the Harley Street nursing home which she supervised shortly before leaving for the Crimea. They show the writer at a relatively little-known period of her life, her character now fully formed, and holding her first responsible job. They portray, too, in stark outline the prevailing social and economic conditions, but above all they reveal her uncanny psychological insight and her underlying humour. These are qualities which must attract the lay reader, but the book will also engage doctors and nurses who still revere Florence Nightingale as the founder of modern hospital practice.

Also by Sir Harry Verney

The Verneys of Claydon

FLORENCE NIGHTINGALE AT HARLEY STREET

Her Reports to the Governors of her Nursing Home
1853—4

with an introduction by Sir Harry Verney, Bt.

H. Verney

London: J. M. Dent & Sons Ltd

Printed in Great Britain by W.P.Griffith & Sons Ltd,
London and Bedford, for
J.M.Dent & Sons Ltd,
Aldine House, Bedford Street, London

ISBN 0 460 03972 5

CONTENTS

Illustrated with manuscript pages from Florence Nightingale's Notebook, and a portrait by her sister Parthenope, between pages 28 and 29

INTRODUCTION

The year 1853 was a milestone, perhaps one of the greatest, in Florence Nightingale's life. She became Superintendent of the Harley Street Nursing Home, her first independent job in nursing, and one which laid the foundations for all that was to follow in her great career.

This post was obtained in the teeth of the fiercest opposition from her family. Her mother, Fanny, 'stormed, lamented and had to be given sal volatile'; her sister Parthe 'wept, raged, worked herself into a frenzy with hysterics, collapsed and had to be put to bed'. Her father wrote sheets in his very difficult handwriting with a quill pen (he abhorred 'great iron spikes') but did nothing.

As Superintendent, Miss Nightingale worked under a Committee of Ladies, presided over by the helpful Lady Canning, who had been instrumental in persuading her to accept the appointment. The other members were elderly, titled well-meaning do-gooders—ladies who in the nursing home had a means of bestowing patronage and charity on the 'lower orders'. Florence Nightingale had one dear friend, Clarkey (Mrs Mohl), to whom she wrote freely and frankly. Clarkey advised her to 'be sure to trample on the Committee and ride the Fashionable Asses rough-shod round Grosvenor Square'. It was a measure of her ability that whilst indeed she trampled on the Committee to obtain what she needed, they never seemed to realize it.

The trouble was this: Could a real Lady accept and obey orders from a Committee of other Ladies; should a 'Lady' nurse someone who was not a Lady? Florence Nightingale could, and did.

Eventually, she went into residence in new premises at 1 Upper Harley Street on 12th August 1853. One of her first difficulties was about religion. The Ladies' Committee had insisted that all patients must be Church of England. She wrote to Clarkey: 'From Committees, charity and schism, from the Church of England, from philanthropy and all deceits of the devil, good Lord deliver us'. 'My Committee refused me to take in Catholic patients; whereupon I wished them good morning, unless I might take in Jews and their Rabbis to attend them.' Miss Nightingale won.

The early days were fraught with difficulties of every kind. In a letter written on 30th August, eighteen days after the opening, she wrote that her father on a visit 'was almost suffocated with gas which went off with a series of partial explosions.

viii

Added to this we had 5 patients dying in the house, the foreman got drunk, and there was a fight between workmen in the drawing room.'

To her father on 4th October 1853 she wrote: 'My dear Papa, between my treasurer who dealt with inexpedient principles and my Committee who dealt with unprincipled expedients, I had a difficult place'.

Then, on 29th October: 'Oh! my boots! my boots! dearer to me than the best French polished. My brother boots! where are my boots! my boots! I ne'er shall see your pretty faces more. My dear, I MUST have them boots. I can't wear your London-made, square-toed, corn begetting rascals.'

Again on 29th October: 'If a repair is not done I will encamp with my twelve patients in the middle of Cavendish Square and let the police and the Committee come and rout me out as a vagrant'.

Within six months all opposition to her ideas had collapsed and on 3rd December 1853 she wrote to her father: 'I am now in the hey-day of my power. Lady—* who was my greatest enemy, is now I understand, trumpeting my fame through London; and all because I have reduced their expenditure from 1/10d. per head per day to 1/-.'

By the spring of 1854 she found time to be gay, and went to parties. She was only 33 and full of fun and a notable mimic. The Nursing Home ran

* Florence Nightingale, perhaps wisely, does not give the lady's name. H.V.

smoothly and gradually she became recognized as a woman of genius.

A short time ago I made an exciting discovery amongst my mother's papers. A very ordinary looking, stiff-bound notebook contained all Florence Nightingale's quarterly reports in her own handwriting, duly signed as Superintendent of the Upper Harley Street Nursing Home. Her Committee are given in minute detail an account of her steward-ship for each of the quarters till she resigned. It was the curtain-raiser for the Crimea.

Here then is the first published copy of this collection of Quarterly Reports to the Ladies' Committee of the Harley Street Nursing Home.

H. Verney

March 1970

November 14. 1853

Sup^t's Quarterly Report
November 14. 1853

As Sup^t, I think it desirable, at the end of three months' service, to make a Report of the State of the Institution to the Ladies' Committee, which I will continue quarterly—stating the changes which I have made during that time.

On the removal of the Institution to Harley St., the linen & furniture were found to be in a most dirty & neglected condition. The table cloths, kitchen cloths, towels, &c, were ragged. There appeared no trace of any mending or darning having been made for many months. The sheets were good. Everything else was rat-eaten. The counterpanes were ragged, & have all been since patched & darned. The towels, though nearly new, had large holes in them. The dusters & the kitchen-cloths were if poſsible, in a worse condition. The blinds were unfit for use, but have been applied to the purpose of lining chair covers. The furniture-covers were unwashed, & the color, in many cases, could hardly be distinguished for dirt. None of these covers were made to take off & on—but were fastened on with tacks (sometimes three deep)—the dirt soaking through. Many nearly new blankets, mattraſses & pillows were spoiled, *even to rotting*, by large stains, owing to having been used (in certain cases) without proper Mackintosh. Vermin ran about tame in all directions.

There have been made (new)

15	prs sheets (linen)
28½	,, pillow-cases
7	dimity bed-furnitures
4	kitchen table-cloths
4	table-cloths, 1½ yds square
18	kitchen-cloths
36	do do
12	dusters
2	Toilet Covers
34	Diaper Towels
64	Check Huckaback Towels
39	green blinds
33	muslin ,,

2 doz. Pincushions & Covers

9 tickings to cover the new spring-beds, which otherwise tear the mattraſses.

These have all been made by Mrs. Clarke, her niece & one house-maid.

The old carpets, which have been cleaned, have been made up afresh at home. The front ward was carpeted anew by Lady Canning, and carpets for three of the attics have been made from the same piece—also at home. Otherwise the old carpets have been sufficient.

The stair-carpets, excepting a few steps at the top, are all made of the old carpets. No more drugget, nor carpeting, nor oil-cloth, nor window-blinds, nor ticking for dividing the rooms will be wanted. There is old curtain sufficient left for this latter purpose.

No charwoman, needlewoman, casual-nurse or night-nurse has been in the house. Since the woman in charge of the house left, 1/6 only has been spent in charing, + 6/10 in needle-work.

Neither has any carpenter's work been wanted, since the carpenters were out of the house.

John has laid down all the carpets, & altered the blinds.

Nurse Smith has helped to piece & join all the carpets, of which not a square inch remains unused.

Nurse Harding has washed many things for the patients, & has helped to make Miſs Robson's outfit for New Zealand, almost the whole of which has been done at home.

viz 3 doz towels
     2 prs sheets
     2 „ pillow cases
    13 diapers
    15 pockethdkfs
besides altering & mending all her clothes.

The furniture & curtains of the Front Ward have been also made entirely at home.

I have thought it desirable to change all the household & the nurses, (more than once)—with the exception of John, the cook, and Nurse Smith. The house has not now the advantage of efficient cleaning—the housemaids being two inexperienced girls, who, though willing and anxious to do all in their power, are unequal to their work without constant superintendence—& therefore more has fallen upon Mrs. Clarke.

I have but three nurses—with whom I am perfectly satisfied—one to each floor. They have had 15 patients among them, & among these, operation & other heavy cases. I have diminished the household by one, having dismifsed the Nurses' Afsistant.

Up to the present time, I have been unable to carry out the rules I could wish, for want of the proper stoves & store-rooms on each floor.

The kitchen-utensils were deficient, no preserving-pan, no saucepan for steaming potatos, no dust-pan, no brushes, no brooms. As much as £2 worth of preserves at one time were had from the Grocer's, as may be seen by the books, at a cost of 1/ p^r pot, & no biscuits were baked at home.

For the sake of securing economy & wholesome bread, I have thought it desirable to bake at home, both bread, biscuits & gingerbread. We bake about 4 stone flour per week for 25 or 26 persons.

4

The preserving is also done at home. We have preserved 52 pots at a cost of 3d½ p^r pot.

I have carried into effect the rule of the patients taking their meals together. From 10-12 dine downstairs every day.

I have made a small alteration about the Servants' washing. All the new nurses & servants are now washed-for by the House-Washerwoman at a cost of 1/ per week, instead of, as formerly, receiving 1/6 per week in money for this purpose.

I have thought it, also, desirable to change some of the Trades people—it having been the custom, as may be seen by the books, to have in articles by the oz. & the half oz—the Grocer's man frequently coming to the house as many as three times a day.

I now lay in groceries *monthly* from Fortnum & Mason's,

flour by the sack from Rymer's,

potatos   d⁰   Covent Garden Market,

apples & onions   d⁰   d⁰

candles by the 4 doz lbs from Davies's

soap   d⁰   d⁰

thereby making the saving between wholesale & retail prices.

On my first entrance, I found scarcely ¼ oz. of stores of any kind in the house.

I have made contracts for

butter at 1/2   pr lb

eggs   1/   for 16

cheese	8d	pr lb
bacon	8d½	pr lb
poultry	4/6	pr couple
meat	7d	pr lb
potatos	13/6	pr sack

the existing prices of provisions being

butter	1/4	pr lb
eggs	1/2	pr doz.
cheese	9d	pr lb
bacon	/9d to /10d pr lb	
poultry	7/ to 9/ pr couple	
meat	/8 to /9 pr lb	
potatos	1d½ per lb	
& bread	10d½ the quartern loaf	

The above prices are therefore lefs than those by which provisions could otherwise be obtained.

The average cost of each person pr day for the last two weeks has been, as may be seen by the books, only 1/ & 1/0½.

Finding a little more light-reading desired by the patients, I take in the "Times", & subscribe to Mudie's for them, but not at the expence of the Institution.

Florence Nightingale
Sup^t.

P.S.

Accommodation for twenty-seven patients is now prepared

6

viz.   10   single rooms
      17   compartments
      ——
      27
      ==

Eighteen patients have been admitted during this quarter

viz.   8   guinea   patients
      10   half guinea   „
      ——
      18
      ==

Of these, 13 are still in the house
           5 have left
Of these five,

1 considerably benefited, (the Case being an incurable one), is now wishing to return (Internal Tumour)

1 discharged as unfit for the Institution (Chronic Rheumatism)

1 benefited (Central Amaurosis)

1 completely cured by an Operation (Cancer of the breast)

1 completely cured by the prospect of New Zealand (Weakneſs)

The whole of the furniture, (including chamber china), of the Front Ward, is new, & has been given by Lady Canning, Mrs. Gilbert & Lady Cranworth. It will accommodate five patients.

Of new furniture procured for the enlarged Institution, the following is the list

    7 bedsteads with mattraſses &c
    3 chests drawers
    4 mats   3 small d°
    6 sofa-cushions
    1 looking-glaſs (secondhand)
    6 chairs
    1 horse
    2 sofas   (second-hand)
    4 tables (,,   ,,)
    3 chairs (,,   ,,)
    3 blankets
    3 counterpanes
  18 rugs

Of *iron-mongery* I have had

    7 fenders
    6 sets fire-irons
    6 door porters
    1 plate-warmer
    2 kettles
    6 coal-scuttles
  12 hearth-brushes
    1 tea-pot

Of *china & glaſs* we have procured

    4 breakfast & tea services for the four floors
  18 divided dishes
    3 sets chamber-china

6 candlesticks
6 flat   d^o
6 small decanters (3 wineglaſs-fuls)
12 tumblers
12 wine glaſses
& a few articles to make up odd sets

The remaining furniture, glaſs & china is all from Chandos St,

Of *what will still be wanted*
8 chairs
4 looking-glaſses
5 washing-stands
5 round tables
3 sofas
1 dreſsing-table
1 nurse's table

are all that are now required to make the accommodation for 27 patients complete. These may be procured second-hand at a small expence.

F.N.

February 20. 1854

2nd Quarterly Report

February 20. 1854

Twenty-seven Patients have been admitted during this Quarter

    viz. 12 guinea Patients

          15 half-guinea „

          ——

          27

          =

Of these, 16 are still in the house

          11 have left

Of these 11,

    1 cured—went to a Situation.

    1 had nothing but idleneſs the matter

    1 left from fear of a slight Operation

    1 *physically* in the same state *morally* worse

    1 cured as far as waywardneſs would allow

    1 improved—left to await the time when an Operation would be desirable

    1 improved—returned to her situation

2 left for Torquay
  (of whom 1 in a hopeleſs state
         1 greatly improved by being discharged)

1 imbecile & not likely to have a return of Sense
1 was brought to the Institution in a state of mental depreſsion, arising immediately from feverishneſs. She required decided medical treatment, by which the cause of her illneſs was, in great measure, removed. At her sister's request she went home, & is now able to occupy herself in her sister's family. In no case, during my knowledge of the Institution, has so much good been done, bodily and mentally, as to this poor Governeſs.

Of those now in the house
  3 cases are waiting for death
    of whom 1 has been here 14 months
         1   8 ,,
         1   3 weeks

To these the house has been an incalculable benefit—miracles of Medical Science, they have benefited still more morally
  3 cases are being rapidly cured of obstinate skin disease
  1 of self-mismanagement
  2 are greatly benefiting

7 are either trifling, hysterical or incurable cases.

―

16

=

It is therefore concluded that

I Of the Patients admitted during the last six months

$\frac{4}{12}$ have derived the greatest benefit

$\frac{3}{12}$ neither good nor harm

$\frac{5}{12}$ have manifestly deteriorated morally & medically

II A Hospital is good for the seriously ill alone— otherwise it becomes a lodging-house where the nervous become more nervous, the foolish more foolish, the idle & selfish more selfish & idle
For two of the elements efsential to a Hospital are *want of occupation* &
directing the attention to bodily health

III There is not a trick in the whole legerdemain of Hysteria which has not been played in this house.

IV On Sundays & Thursdays, patients prepare themselves for the Ladies' Committee & the Medical Men—exactly as Roman Catholic women do for confefsion—by getting up a case. It is dull to be always saying the same thing. Therefore some patients leave off their flannels on Sunday in order to have a cough for Monday. I have known a patient, so hungry as to steal another patient's meal, who yet left all her own meals untasted (in order to prove her want of appetite) & ate them in the night.

V The family tie is so strong as to induce the best to keep their sick at home, unlefs there be something in the character of these sick which impels the family to try to get rid of the burden. This feeling, first, &, secondly, the fear of the *so-called* degradation of a Public Institution produce—as a consequence natural & to be expected—that (for many years at least) such an Institution as this will have, as Patients

1 those who have wearied out their families, or been wearied out by them

2 those who have no families at all

3 wives or daughters, anxious to return to their families & to save them expence

In this Institution, the families of, at least, $\frac{7}{12}$ of the Patients have come to me & said "*Now you know her,* you see we *could* not keep her at home"

Conclusion—that, if the Medical Certificate be not strictly enforced, this will become, not a Hospital for the Sick, but a Hospital for incompatible tempers & for hysterical fancies.

VI *Gentility* & *eating* & *drinking* (more particularly

drinking, wine or spirits) are two of the main subjects of interest.

VII Where there is no higher interest in life, illnefs naturally becomes an amusement & a luxury. If nothing occupies a woman more than her dinner & her mucous membrane, her mucous membrane & her dinner will become her sole object—to breakfast in bed & to be pitied her sole solace.

Unmitigated harm is done, in such cases, by visiting, where the Visitor makes the comforts of the Patient the chief topic. And the efforts for a month of the Doctor & attendants to throw the patient's thoughts away from herself may be undone by a Visitor in one $\frac{1}{4}$ hour. Such patients *would*, at any time, be well, *if they would*.

These cases are always aggravated in a Hospital.

VIII To fit a patient *for life*, if they are to live (as well as for death, if they are to die) is, it is to be hoped, one of the objects of a Hospital. Here patients are often *un*fitted for life, by being enervated rather than invigorated. The main cause of this is the fallacy of allowing them to believe that their own payments cover their expences. It difsatisfies them with all life after. "It is not like Harley St." "I had such & such for my 10/6 at Harley St."

What is to be done to save such patients from being spoiled?

The housekeeping expences cannot be further

reduced. They are now barely more than 1/ a day per head.

The attendance cannot be further reduced. There are now two nurses only to 17 patients, 6 of whom are very heavy cases.

The furniture *is there* & must be taken care of.

It would appear that the only thing which can now be done is to limit the cases to those of *real* illnefs.

IX Of the half-guinea Patients, admitted during the last six months, four only, out of seventeen, have been real "*Hospital*" cases. Thirteen have been put in here by their friends (or their protectors) as a temporary Asylum, some of whom have upbraided us for its not being a permanent one. It is a curious pathological fact that such Patients always take to their bed on the third day after their admifsion.

X The main things (as far as I have had experience in this matter) to be asked of the Ladies' Committee are

1. to limit the admifsions to cases of serious illnefs.

2. to take other cases *on approval* only for a week or a fortnight, with the condition that they then depart, if the Medical Officers declare them unlikely to benefit by medical treatment

3. to administer strictly the rule, which already

exists, that Patients be limited, as to their stay, to a period of two months, & that they consider it as being so limited unlefs in cases, which the Medical Men will specify, where recovery or death is anticipated.

4. to entreat the help of the Lady Visitors to afsist the Medical Men & attendants in turning the attention of the Patients *out of* themselves & their comforts

5. to further the efforts of discharged Patients to find occupations.

Our Quarter's work has been

(1) darning, mending & turning the old sheets, darning & mending the old pillow-cases & towels, darning quilts & blankets

(2) making up the old kitchen-cloths into dusters & basin-cloths by doubling them—for they were rotten—& fragments of the old chintz & old pantry-cloths into dusters. Making these into sets for each of the 4 floors, marked A, B, C & D so as to keep the floors separate.

(3) as, upon most of the furniture, there were covers, three deep, fastened with *tacks,* we have taken all these off, washed them, patched them and lined them & made them up into covers, so that there are now two, at least, for each piece of furniture (to change)

(4) we have new-covered the drawing-room furniture, lining it all with the new blue chintz

(5) made chair-covers out of the old striped curtains,
4 sofa-covers out of different old pieces (also lined).
We have required 12 y^{ds} only of new lining, the old
blinds from Chandos St. having served as for lining
(6) made 3 new dimity bed-furnitures
   2 new ticking chair-covers
 finished the new sheets & pillow-cases
All this work has been done in the house.
We have spent 5/6 in charing
     o in needlework
     o in night-nursing
during this Quarter.
 We have had 6 new blankets
    1 door mat
  also 1 doz. deſsert spoons, electro-plated
   1 doz. tea   ,, ,,
   1 doz. small knives & forks ,,
   3 sieves
  also 6 broth-basins
   6 mugs
   1 candle-stick

       Florence Nightingale
        Sup^t.

May 15. 1854

3rd Quarterly Report
May 15. 1854

There have been 30 Patients in the Institution during this Quarter
   viz. 18 guinea Patients
      12 half-guinea „
      ——
      30
      =

Of these, 9 are still in the House
        21 have left

Of these 21
  3 cured by Operation
    (2 completely
    1 as far as disease admitted)
    returned to their homes & have since re-
    peatedly written to tell of their well-being
  3 cured entirely of obstinate skin-diseases
  1 cured of long-standing disease
  1   of self-mismanagement
    This was a case which a Homoeopathic

quack would have cried about the streets with a portrait. She came to us, having been confined to her bed for 3 years, & believing herself incapable of taking solid food or anything but Port Wine & cream. She left us, (in two months) restored to the use of her feet & her senses, eating meat & taking long walks like other people. But this could only have been done by isolating her from the other patients & from *all* influences which would have strengthened her illusions. She was cured, almost without a grain of medicine.

1 greatly benefited, left for a situation after a year's residence in the Institution.

1 somewhat improved, left for the Brompton Hospital

2 left incurable after having been here 5 and 6 months

3 hysterical—no improvement

2 died

The benefits which this Institution ought to afford to the sick are perhaps best seen when we are enabled to give comfort in the time of danger & to lefsen the agony of death. In no case, which we have had under our care, was the value of the Institution so evident as in that of a friendlefs foreigner, dying in a Public Hospital, who was brought here. At the first visit, the Physician pronounced her to be actually dying. The contest between life & death, usually so short, was however protracted to no less than 5 days. During this time, her fearful sufferings required constant medical treatment, by which the most dreadful kind of death was, at least at intervals, freed from pain, & even a smile, from time to time, rewarded those who were around her, to whom, when afsured of their sympathy, she was able to exprefs her thoughts & feelings.

4 left, cured of complaints which never existed— their individual objects having been obtained

  viz. 1 of finding a situation
    1 of making Pomade
    2 of finding here a comfortable lodging-house

One of these had been in the Institution during the last month. On admifsion she stated that she was too ill to move, or indeed to do anything except to mourn over her misfortunes & to eat & to drink. The physician found only weaknefs & slight cough. Her complaint, in fact, was the result of her circumstances & consisted chiefly in lofs of energy & will to exert herself. She was soon induced to get up & to walk out, and it was very apparent that she wanted no medical treatment but only hopeful occupation, which unfortunately is not to be obtained in an Institution of this kind.

Of the 9 now in the house
  2 are still awaiting their departure out of this world

1 is being cured of a skin disease
1 recovering from an Operation
1 awaiting one
2 are eye cases
1 is in a hopeleſs state of Consumption
1 slowly improving—(Hysteria

I have carried out the rule that the Superintendent shall attend the Doctors' visits, in every case but one; experience having proved the impoſsibility of conducting this or any similar Institution where such attendance is not rigidly adhered to. In that one case, I have *as yet* waived the rule, at her expreſs desire (she being an old Patient from Chandos St, where unfortunately it had never been enforced). Experience of the results of the *exception* has fully justified the rule. The mistakes which have arisen have been Legion—directions misunderstood, or not given at all, or forgotten. Rather than permit such exceptions in future, it would be consistent that the Superintendent should resign an impoſsible position (viz. that of undertaking to execute orders which she never hears, except as represented by the Patients) such position being incompatible with the good order of the house & her duty to the Institution.

There have been admitted many cases which proved to be unworthy of the Charity—&, in such, the disastrous effects of indiscriminate visiting have been plainly manifested. It is due to the Committee conscientiously to reiterate the result of experience, viz. that the visits of neither Chaplain nor Lady Visitors can be efficaciously made without previous conference with those who alone can be aware of the medical & moral state of each Patient—it being obvious that, otherwise, such visits are like those of a Medical Man who should be ignorant of the diagnosis of his Patient.

I would call the attention of the Committee to the fact that, for the last two months, the number of Patients in the house has not averaged more than nine. As it is much more economical to provide for nine & twenty than for nine, I have lately had the greater difficulty in maintaining the average cost per head of each person in the house at so low a rate as 1/ or 1/2 per day. And even with this low average, the Patients' Payments have not covered the house-keeping expences. These will, again, be higher, because, owing to the increased price of meat, the butcher has refused to continue the contract which I made when I first entered nine months ago, viz. to furnish all meat at /7 pr lb, & I am now compelled to give /7½. The fact of the deficiency of Patients calls for immediate attention. Otherwise, this Institution will degenerate into a luxurious piece of charity, not worth burthening the public with. The expences now amount to £1500 pr an—the Receipts, including Subscriptions & Patients' Payments, to leſs than £1000 pr an. The Donations have all been swallowed up in covering the building & other extra expenditure of last year.

I have changed one housemaid, on account of her love of dirt and inexperience, & one nurse, on account of her love of Opium & intimidation.

We have had much illneſs in the household, but all have been found willing to help one another. We have spent
   2/3 in charing
   o   in needlework
   o   in night nursing
      or casual nursing
altho' we have had two deaths & four operations.

Our quarter's work has been
(1) finishing the Drawing-Room furniture
(2) making 5 sofa-covers out of old material & lining them; in order that all the bed-room sofas may also have two covers apiece
(3) making 2 ticking arm-chair covers
         2   d°
         one of the old blue striped curtains, which have now made five. The old red curtains have made six. There are now covers enough to change all the arm-chairs.

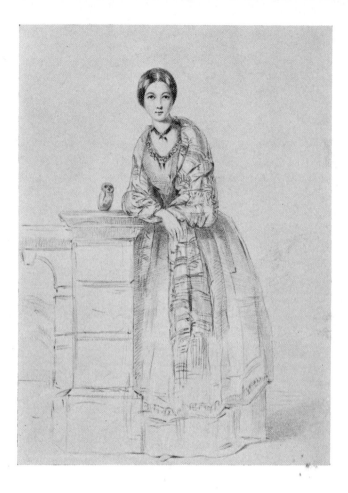

Florence Nightingale

from a portrait by her sister Parthenope

I have carried out the rule that
the Superintendent shall attend the
Doctors' visits, in every case but one;
experience having proved the impossibility
of conducting this or any similar
Institution where such attendance is
not rigidly adhered to. In that one
case, I have as yet waived the rule,
at her express desire (she being an
old Patient from Chandos St, where
unfortunately it had never been enforced)
Experience of the results of the exception
has fully justified the rule. The
mistakes which have arisen have
been legion — directions Misunderstood,
or not given at all, or forgotten.
Rather than permit such exceptions
in future, it would be consistent
that the Superintendent should resign
an impossible position (viz. that of
undertaking to execute orders which
she never hears, except as represented

Institution will degenerate into a luxurious piece of charity, not worth burthening the public with. The expences now amount to £1500 pr an — the Receipts, including Subscriptions & Patients' Payments, to less than £1000 pr an. The Donations have all been swallowed up in covering the building & other extra expenditure of last year.

I have changed one housemaid, on account of her love of dirt and inexperience — & one nurse, on account of her love of Opium & intimidation —

We have had much illness in the household, but all have been found willing to help one another. We have spent

2/3	in	charing
0	in	Needle work
0	in	Night Nursing
	on	casual nursing

altho' we have had two deaths & four operations.

& economy, the result has been to me most satisfactory.

I therefore wish, at the close of the year for which I promised my services, to intimate that,—having, as I believe, done the work as far as it can be done,—it is probable that I may retire, if, in pursuance of my design & the allegiance which I hold to it, I meet with a sphere which is more analogous to the formation of a Nursing School.

I would wish to give a notice of three months, to be extended, if possible, to six months

I have made these explanations, feeling that I am in honor bound clearly to explain to the Ladies' Committee, at the end of the year, the conclusions to which I have come with regard to the Institution in which we are all so much interested.

Florence Nightingale
Supt.

(4) making 1 doz. dusters
    2 table-cloths
    8 toilet-covers
    4 sand-bags (old green baize
    2 Anti-Macaſsars
  making old print into dusters
  doubling old towels into cloths
  cleaning & mending carpets
  repairing counterpanes
     pillow-cases
     towels

As it appeared to have been customary in this Institution, when an article of furniture was dirty, to tack a new piece of Chintz over it, & when an article of bed-clothing had a hole in it, to let such hole continue till a new one was to be bought, I have been thus minute in recording the progreſs of the mysteries of making & mending, in order to account for the stores of old rags which came under my charge when I entered into service here.

We have had 1 piece calico for lining.

Florence Nightingale
Sup^t.

August 7. 1854

4th Quarterly Report

August 7. 1854

Twenty-two Patients have been in the Institution
during this quarter
   viz.   9 guinea Patients
       13 half-guinea   ,,

Of these, 10 are still in the house
          12 have left

Of these 12
- 1 (Consumption, from the first, hopelefs) left, considerably relieved, for the sea-side, after 4 months.
- 1 (eye-case) slightly relieved
- 2 (Operations) cured
- 3 (Hysteria—Skin disease—Mucous Membrane) cured
- 2 greatly relieved
- 1 (Cataract) operated upon—eye lost, by inflammation supervening.
- 1 improved as far as 72 years admitted

1 admitted only to attend her child during an Operation, departed, leaving the child here.

Of the 10 now in the house

    5 without hope of recovery, are awaiting their end at periods varying from a few days to many months

    2 fancy-Patients

    1 a child recovering from an Operation

    1 spine case

    1 moral case

There have been 4 Operations.

The Nº of Patients in the house at once has varied from 5 to 13 during this quarter.

There have been 60 Patients during the *Year*.

We have made 3 sofa-covers

            2 night-caps

have repaired the linen

            2 haſsocks.

We have preserved

        30 pots Red Currant Jam

        6 ,,   ,,   ,, Jelly

at a cost of /2d per pot

We have had but one nurse for some time, the other nurse having been taken ill & sent into the country to recover.

We have spent 7/6 in casual nursing

        0   in night   ,,

        0   in charing

        0   in needle work

We have saved half the Afsistant Medical Officer's salary by dispensing at home, which has also considerably reduced our account at Savory & Moore's.

The wages paid during this Quarter have been lefs by £9 than those paid during the last Quarter.

The year having now expired, for which I undertook the office of Sup^t of this Institution, the Ladies' Committee will naturally expect that I should give some notice to them of my views as to our succefs.

I would wish therefore to exprefs that I consider my work is now done, & that the Institution has been brought into as good a state as its capabilities admit.

I have not effected anything towards the object of training nurses—my primary idea in devoting my life to Hospital work for, owing to the small number of applications, the Committee have not been able to select, in all cases, proper objects for Medical & Surgical treatment—and accordingly the result has not been satisfactory to me.

In every other respect, viz. as to good order, good nursing, moral influence & economy, the result has been to me most satisfactory.

I therefore wish, at the close of the year for which I promised my services, to intimate that,—having, as I believe, done the work *as far as it can be done,*—it is probable that I may retire, *if,* in pursuance of my design & the allegiance which I hold to it, I meet with a sphere which is more analogous to the formation of a Nursing School.

I would wish to give a notice of three months, to be extended, if pofsible, to six months.

I have made these explanations, feeling that I am in honor bound clearly to explain to the Ladies' Committee, at the end of the year, the conclusions to which I have come with regard to the Institution in which we are all so much interested.

Florence Nightingale
Sup^t.